CHAPTER ONE: INTRO

The 500 solution is a unique mental-state approach to weight loss and a healthy lifestyle.

Stop spending money on workout programs that won't work for you. All the information you need is out there. It's all free and all available.

There are 10 basic choices that you make daily.

After you make 500 of these choices in a row you will have burned away most of your excess body fat. It's that simple.

The 500 Solution will walk you through how to get there.

- What mindset to take.

- How to be decisive, recognizing that most of the perceived difficulty in these choices is your mindset.

- Understanding that indecision leads to failure.

- You will decide at each moment and with each decision your willpower grows stronger and your results will speak for themselves.

- You will still be able to eat your favourite treats and foods, in moderation, through a rewards system!

People will ask what your secret is and that's when you'll realize that *there is no secret*. We all know what to do and how to eat; it's your mindset that changes everything forever.

Everybody is different. Every diet is different. This isn't about what to eat, it's about how to think about eating. The biggest hurdle to weight loss and a fitter body isn't lack of knowledge. You can learn just about anything about diets and nutrition. It's all about finding what works for you through trial-and-error and creating consistency.

Emerging research is starting to indicate that nutrition is actually much more individualistic than we think. For instance, something as simple as what age you were when you took antibiotics could affect, on a cellular level, how you metabolize complex carbohydrates. That's why some people swear by diets that seem to do nothing for you!

That being said, there are simple choices you can make within the 500 Solution that guarantee success.

- Cut out sugar

- Cut out fast food

- Cut out junk carbohydrates

Following those 3 laws consistently through time will guarantee you weight loss. So why not start there?

Building muscle, growing lean mass and any other fitness goals you might have can happen *after* the 500. Start with nutrition. Start with one brick to build a wall.

But you already know this. If you eat well and then also workout, that's all it takes to succeed. That's the secret. Most people do that only 1 or 2 days a week. The other people, the ones we follow on Instagram and buy their workout programs and hate on the beach in August, they do it *all the time.* And guess what? They don't understand why everyone isn't doing it. It's easy. You're eating anyways, just eat something different. You're watching Netflix, just jog for 20 minutes instead. You don't have a spare 20 minutes? You're quite literally the most important and busiest person in the world? Or are you lying to yourself? Are you just making excuses? They may be valid excuses but they don't change the reality of actions and consequences.

You can't walk into a Porsche dealership and say "I only have enough money for a Toyota but you should give me a Porsche anyway because I have all these circumstances in my life that make it hard for me to make more money". The same goes for fitness, you have to earn it.

When you face your 500th moment and make the right choice, the pride you feel will be worth every single step you've taken on this journey. You'll laugh at your old self; *how did that person ever convince me that skipping the gym and eating bad was making me happier than I feel right now?*

You'll be awake for the first time in a long time. And you'll feel so damn good. Everything in life will just seem easier because your mind has changed. You can see that this principle of *action + time = results* can relate to everything you do. You'll also realize that the only reason you hated people in shape and made fun of people who went to gyms is because of your own insecurities and unhappiness. No one can be truly happy when they know they aren't being the best person they can be.

When you're staring at your 500th moment, you'll realize that you're happier than you could have imagined. You'll feel so proud. In only 50 days none of your clothes will fit anymore; they'll all be too big! Your only negative thought will be '*why the hell didn't I do this years ago*'.

CHAPTER TWO: THE MOMENTS

There are 10 decision-moments you will face every single day. So the first thing we need to do is to identify those key moments.

1. Exercise. Are you listing all the reasons you don't have time to work-out? Have you

convinced yourself that it doesn't make sense to exercise today? Are you planning to skip today but workout tomorrow? These are conscious choices. If you decide not to exercise because of any of these excuses then you are lying to yourself.

2. Breakfast. What to eat for breakfast/ choosing to eat breakfast

3. AM Snack. The mid-morning snack we need to get through to lunch.

4. Lunch. What are you going to eat?

5. PM Snack. Are you eating because it's something to do? Are you wanting to reward

    yourself? Are you going to eat a treat? Are you eating to cheer yourself up? All of that is ok and totally normal. So what are you going to eat?

6. Appetizers. Feeling a little hungry? Want to pass the time? What are you going to eat?

7. Dinner. What are you going to eat for dinner?

8. Dessert. Choose not to eat a dessert. Don't tell yourself that life is too short to skip something sweet. Life is long, you want to look good and feel good for most of it. Be proud of overcoming these moments.

9. Evening Temptation. You will want to snack. If you made a bad choice on number 1 now is a good time to exercise; if you have time to snack while watching television then you have time to work out. Do anything that gets you moving.

10. Final Snack. Congratulations. You've already made 9 life-changing decisions today. This last one is so important to burn fat. Make a snack from our food list **(See Appendix).** This one can be hard at first but it gets easier.

Imagine 50 days in a row like this; your excess fat is already starting to burn away. You can do it this time. Life going on around you has nothing to do with this; there will always be excuses to choose from. Get your mind right and your body will follow.

That's it. This is how easy it's going to be. 10 decisions you will consciously make every day. You will slip up and that's ok. There will be rewards throughout this process and you'll realize that this is NOT "dieting"; this is just living. You won't miss the crap food and the sugars because we are going to break down your addictions and the cravings that have been imprinted into your subconscious mind.

10 good choices a day. It's that simple. By the time you make 500 good choices in a row, you won't even notice you're doing it anymore. You'll lose so much body fat that you'll find yourself full of energy. You'll want to surround yourself with other positive people who also have the right mindset. Living longer, feeling better, looking great and increasing your self-worth. You are about to become an inspiration for everyone in your life. Own it, love it, and celebrate yourself.

Take a picture of yourself, put your measurements on the back and put that on the fridge. You're never going to be that person again. This. Is. Exciting. This is the moment your entire life changed.

This book provides your Daily Decision List for you to follow and check off. Preparation is key. At the end of this book you'll find a list of great food choices for each decision moment. These are just suggestions to help you get started, find what works for you. Also, check out the end sections about Ketogenetic and Low-carb dieting as well as Intermittent Fasting and Time-Restricted Eating.

Now, let's break down moments 1 – 10 in more detail. I highly recommend getting through this guide before you kick things off so that you have all the tools you need to be successful.

Decision Moment #1 Exercise EVERYDAY. Be ACTIVE every day.

You're going to exercise. And you're going to do it even on the days you really don't want to. You're going to focus on how proud you feel after you workout on those days. You're going to notice that you feel better than you did beforehand and you're going to remember that every time you lie to yourself with all the reasons you can't work out today.

It doesn't matter when you workout. It doesn't matter what you do to workout. Go to a gym and do something. The more you go the more you'll learn and the more you'll try new things.

Decision Moment #2 Breakfast

You just woke up. You're about to set the tone for the entire day. Are you used to a greasy treat? Do you normally have a bagel with cream cheese or some toast with butter and eggs? I know that I love dipping my toast in eggs; it's always one of my reward meals. But the empty carbs, high sugar cereals, breakfast sandwiches, and sugar in your coffee all needs to stop. Not eating breakfast is a choice too. See the section on *Intermittent Fasting*, it may be a good choice for you. If you do eat, eat a 'Fitness Breakfast': A fitness breakfast is like having a shower and putting on clean clothes in the morning. It sets the tone. It's step one. If you venture out in your pyjamas and slippers you're telling the world that you have no intention of taking the day seriously. When you start the day with an unfit food choice you've decided not to take your health seriously.

After you've made this choice only a few times you will be amazed how easy it really is to rewire your brain to this new way of eating in the morning. So much of our morning is on autopilot anyway, just rewrite your rules. Here's an example of how your breakfast decision affects your whole day: You have a breakfast sandwich with sausage and cheese to start your day. Delicious, right? But just moments after eating it you already feel sluggish and bloated. You choose an outfit that reflects that feeling. You're already not your best you and it's not even 9am.

Next, it's time for a mid-morning snack and even though you brought a banana all the sugar in that breakfast sandwich is starting to lose its effect and you are craving something sweet. So instead you have a muffin; what's the difference, you already had a breakfast sandwich, right? And so this goes throughout the day. When you do feel guilty about it you tell yourself that you will start a diet tomorrow or research on the internet about ways to lose weight. You feel better because you have a plan. But a plan is worthless if you're never willing to take that first step.

Fast forward 3 months and you're in the same cycle. Break it. It's time to stop and take the first step.

Cut the bullshit. Start with a fitness breakfast, choice number one. Make it and be proud. Feel good about it.

Break your current breakfast habit and eat smart. Make the right choice. This is your first moment of change. Take it head on with everything you have. Don't forget that you're doing this for you. *Single moments added up over time are what create meaningful change.*

You know that if you eat a burger every day for a year those add up. But if you don't eat that burger every day those add up too, and in a wonderful way! Begin by being proud of yourself for making the right choice in this moment. This is a victory. You have just broken out of a bad habit. Imagine what else you can do.

Decision Moment #3 AM Snack

Let's say you're at work. You had a healthy breakfast, good job! Now let's make that count. Decision Moment 2 or midmorning snack is one of the most difficult moments (at first). The dead period between beginning your day at work and lunchtime can play tricks on you.

You start to tell yourself that a treat will pass the time. That you deserve to eat whatever you want because you had a healthy breakfast or because your day is stressful or because you're bored. Or that everyone else is eating a treat so you can too. It's very simple to find an excuse here.

Make the decision and don't look back: *I'm going to eat a fitness food.*

Even if you succeed in convincing yourself that life isn't worth living without a muffin, force yourself to eat the fitness food FIRST anyway. You'll realize that the act of eating is all you really needed. You got the break you wanted and you'll feel better about yourself for having made that choice. Suddenly you'll realize that the muffin isn't necessary for your happiness after all. In fact, if you measured your happiness minutes after eating the muffin and minutes after eating the fitness food you would notice that you were significantly happier after eating well. So make the right choice, even if everyone around you isn't.

What if you said yes to that muffin instead, as so many people do every single day? Do you really think you can avoid gaining weight if you ate around 200 muffins a year? And for what? A few moments of enjoyment that are fleeting and which eventually turn to disdain. It's a moment that can be filled by a food that actually helps you LOSE fat, instead of gain it. Start making new choices. Be the inspiration in your own life. People will try to make you fail because your success magnifies their own bad choices. Don't listen. In a few short weeks they are going to see how all these little choices, one by one, added up to big changes. Just a few weeks. One little moment at a time. Let them make jokes about you being a health nut or whatever it is they say to project their own insecurities onto you. Just smile and know that your life is different now. This is your story and this is the part where you reinvent yourself

Decision Moment #4 Lunch

Finally, lunchtime. You were good and made your lunch the night before but now all you want is to treat yourself. Maybe your friends are going out for lunch or you're fantasizing about getting a sandwich or pizza or something along those lines because you're hungry and no one wants healthy food when they're famished, right?

It's decision time. This is a moment. Chose right here. You'll be happy that you did. Not only will you be choosing to lose extra fat but you'll also be choosing to feel good for the rest of the day. Who needs that awful heavy feeling all afternoon after a greasy indulgence?

No matter what, eat the lunch that you brought. Once you satisfy your actual hunger, your subconscious desire to eat something bad for you will weaken.

That's 4 moments today. Four moments that normally lead to weight gain over time. Pay attention to how you feel after lunch. Be proud of yourself. You aren't depriving yourself of anything. You're eating the way humans are meant to eat; to maximize your output and caloric burn and to sustain positive energy levels.

Decision Moment #5 PM Snack

The dreaded afternoon lull.

This is a tough one. It's that 3pm moment when something sweet sounds way too good to pass up. But here's the thing; if you don't pass it up today you probably won't pass it up tomorrow. Don't envy your co-worker who claims "not to care". That one bad decision becomes 5 bad decisions becomes 50 becomes 1,000. Be strong. *Eat.* By all means eat. But eat smart and with fitness and your goals in mind. Every moment is a choice and if making the right choice was easy, then everyone would do it all the time. But they don't, because change is difficult. You're better than them.

Don't let yourself make excuses for bad decisions. With every choice, you're getting fit, healthier and losing fat. It's happening, let it. All you need to do is choose this moment.

Decision Moment #6 Appetizer

For most of us there's a dead period after our work day is done and before dinner is ready. Perhaps it's going to take an hour to cook or you need groceries first or you're going out for dinner so you're eating later than normal. In any circumstance, you will want to snack before dinner. This is especially true if you've exercised already today. Your body will be craving carbs and trying to coerce your mind into giving in to all temptation.

This moment is a decision without a substitute. *Choose not to eat anything.* The health shake/food you had directly after working out was enough and if you haven't worked out yet then you definitely don't need anything. It only takes a couple days in a row of making this choice for this particular craving to disappear.

You'll enjoy your dinner a lot more as well.

Decision Moment #7 Dinner

This is an easy one once you decide to make fitness meals. Get the idea of ordering take-out food out of your head. It's not an option and it's actually a myth that it's cheaper; check out our dinner grocery lists **(See Appendix)** for proof of that. *Have a big hearty dinner.* It will help you from snacking later.

You didn't make good choices all day just to order a pizza now, did you? How many times are you going to make the same mistakes? You know that you will be happy at first if you order in food. When it comes it smells so good and it's warm and you sit down and eat. But afterwards you quickly start to regret that choice; you're too full and you feel fat and you're ashamed that you gave in to your craving. We've all been there many, many times. Stop making the wrong choice.

Plus, an hour after eating you'll be hungry again and since you already ate pizza and hate yourself you figure you may as well eat chips. Fast forward six months and you've been in a shame eating spiral and gained another 10lbs of fat. That bullshit stops now. Enough is enough. Get smart. You're reading this because you're ready to be done with that bullshit cycle. This is the time to reinvent yourself. These small moments, these are what will define your future self.

Decision Moment #8 Dessert

It's 5 to 10 minutes after dinner. This is a very real moment. You want to be able to keep eating; something sweet would really hit the spot. Repeat this to yourself: "This is a craving. *I'm not going to eat right now, like it or not*" and then find a distraction. You'll eat in a couple of hours anyway, it won't kill you to wait. Be proud of yourself when you do this, it's a difficult moment to win. But it's also one of the easiest to get used to. You won't even notice this moment after a few days, I promise.

Decision Moment #9 Evening Temptation

About an hour after dinner most people are starting to shut down for the night. For most of us that means some quality TV time. *Try watching TV without a snack.* Decision Moments 9 and 10 can be interchanged so if you do decide to have a snack here, have a smart one. Sugars and empty carbs at this time will spend all night converting into fat.

Also, if you haven't worked out yet, look at what you're doing right now. Look at how many hours are left before you go to bed. Is there time to go to a gym? Can you do jumping jacks or push-ups in your bedroom? How about some yoga? I'm willing to bet there is time for that.

Choose that. Choose to pack up some gym clothes. Then choose that you're going to go to your car or walk to the bus stop. Then, no matter what, get changed at the gym. You'll exercise if you do that, I promise. And you'll feel amazing. And what's more, you didn't just spend that time eating chips in front of the TV!

Go home and have a fitness snack and some TV time; now, you've earned it!

Decision Moment #10 THE LONG GOODNIGHT

You'll eat at night. There's no way around it. It's how we're wired and we want your health and fitness lifestyle to be realistic. Just start seeing your food options differently. Don't obsess over chips or ice cream or whatever your weakness happens to be. When those thoughts pop into your head, shoo them away and tell yourself 'I've decided to change. Chips (or whatever) are not even an option".

It's indecision that causes our self-torture. *I want chips but I can't have them. Should I get pizza tonight? Should I go to the gym?* Destroy indecision by eliminating options. Eating junk is just not an option anymore. Done.

We always come up with great reasons to get the answers we want to make the decisions that we know are bad ones.

CHAPTER 3: THE PROGRAM

Here's How It Works:

There are 3 levels

- Level 1 is passing 10 moments in a row.
- Level 2 is 50 moments in a row.
    - ✓ Level 2 has 1 reward.
- Level 3 is passing 500 moments in a row.
    - ✓ Level 3 includes 5 rewards.

The Rewards

Once you get through half of Level 2 (25 moments) you can claim a reward for yourself for any day within those 5 days.

Once you hit 100 moments you get a reward point and will get another reward point for every 100 moments you pass following that.

So, in other words, you are still going to be able to enjoy your favourite foods because life is all about moderation, and this system is designed to be a new way of eating for the rest of your life.

Write down what your reward meals or snacks are going to be. That way you always have something to look forward to, especially during those difficult moments where you try to convince yourself to give up.

Here's an example:

After I hit 5 days in a row I'm going to order a pizza for dinner on day 6.

After that, I'll go 10 days in a row (100 moments), and then have chocolate cake for dessert on day 11. Following the next 10 days in a row, I'm going to have a big breakfast of pancakes and bacon on Day 26. And this goes on. Most likely, you'll be feeling and looking so good that may not even bother with the rewards. But they're there to keep you motivated and moving!

Reward food is so much tastier and fulfilling when it's earned. Somewhere over the past 50-60 years we all forgot that these foods were meant as a treat, not as a replacement for our day-to-day nutritional fulfilment.

This is the secret to eating cake and not feeling guilty!

CHAPTER 4: TRACKING YOUR PROGRESS

You will go through ups and downs emotionally. Sometimes it will feel like you're not losing any weight and this is all useless. It's not. Every donut you choose to eat adds up and every donut you choose NOT to eat adds up. So it's important to track. Never let failures stop you from moving forward; we all fail sometimes. Those who succeed are the ones who dust themselves off and keep going.

TRACKING HELP

Here's what you need to do; fill out the info below and look at the numbers every 10 days that you follow the program. This is so very important because there will be times when you feel like this is all for nothing because you think you're not losing any weight or fat. But you are. Trust in this and believe in yourself.

Be ready for this: One week your weight will drop, the next you may gain weight...and so on. Trust the process and stick with it. The ups and downs are part of it. Everyone else quits; not you, not this time. This time let's see what happens when you don't give up.

DAY ONE

Weight ________________

BMI   ________________

Fat %   ______________

Pick one outfit that you will put on at Moment 500

Track every 10 days

DAY TEN

Weight ________________

BMI   ________________

Fat %   ______________

Pick one outfit that you will put on every 10 days.

DAY TWENTY

Weight ________________

BMI   ________________

Fat %   ______________

DAY THIRTY

Weight ________________

BMI ___________________

Fat % ______________

DAY FORTY

Weight ________________

BMI ___________________

Fat % ______________

DAY FIFTY- MOMENT 500!

Weight ________________

BMI ___________________

Fat % ______________

Put on the outfit from DAY ONE

Success Tracker

Use the following template to track yourself as you get
started. It's very common for people to take 2 or 3 tries
before getting through the first 10 moments. But, once
you do the first 10, that moment of revelation, where you
did it, you will feel a euphoria wash over you as the
realization that this *is possible* and that you're going to
success this time becomes reality!

Daily Moments

- Moment 1 Success! I worked out!

  ____

  ____

- Moment 1 Fail. I did nothing active and instead

  I____

- Moment 2 Success! I ate

  ____

  ____

- Moment 2 Fail. I ate

  ____

  ____

- Moment 3 Success! I ate

  ____

  ____

- Moment 3 Fail. I ate

  ____

  ____

- Moment 4 Success! I ate____

  ____

- Moment 4 Fail. I ate

  ____

  ____

- Moment 5 Success! I ate____

  ____

- Moment 5 Fail. I ate

  ____

  ____

- Moment 6 Success! I ate

  ____

  ____

- Moment 6 Fail. I ate

  ____

  ____

- Moment 7 Success! I ate

  ____

  ____

- Moment 7 Fail. I ate

  ____

  ____

- Moment 8 Success! I ate____

  ____

- Moment 8 Fail. I ate

  ____

  ____

- Moment 9 Success! I ate____

  ____

- Moment 9 Fail. I ate

  ____

  ____

- Moment 10 Success! I ate

  ____

  ____

- Moment 10 Fail. I ate

  ____

  ____

There are so many reasons to fail these moments. It's really important to focus on each successful moment and to be proud of yourself.

I've worked with thousands of people and the successful ones all have the same revelation:

It's amazing, I've spent my whole life struggling with not eating well and craving foods that are bad for me. The first 10 moments were so much harder than the final 500. And after the first 100, it wasn't even difficult at all. It's just those first few days...

That's the really amazing part of this journey: there's no magic pill or crazy diet. The secret lies in realizing that you just need to make a good choice about 10 times per day. One day at a time and your body begins to change. It's much more addicting than any food will ever be. Trust the process.

We are always expecting immediate results. You won't get immediate results in the appearance of your body. That will happen over time. Trust the process.

But you WILL get immediate results in your mental blueprint that maps how you approach food and life. Again, be proud of yourself for every moment you win! This is one moment...imagine 500 more like these and inches of fat just gone!

I've heard every excuse, every reason, and every logical argument for failing these moments. And they're all real, they're all valid. But that doesn't change the results of that kind of thinking.   You can't convince your body not to convert sugars into fat because you're having a bad day, or you're bored, or you've earned a treat. Your body doesn't care; it has a job to do and will adapt based on what you put in it.

So here's what we tell ourselves:

What's the point of living if you can't be happy?

Really? Tell me how happy you are 5 minutes AFTER you eat that garbage. Start experiencing real and long term happiness, not these temporary fixes that cause extreme unhappiness and shame afterwards. 500 moments from now, ask yourself if you'd be happier if you had spent the last month eating all that crap.

You're an adult, stop eating treats and acting as though life fulfillment comes from ice cream. Be better than that. Rise above that. Become the better version of yourself that you know you can be.

Well, fuck it, I already ate the (blank) so what's the difference if I eat (blank)?

Let's say you own a gym. A membership only costs $10 per month. So one person comes in and wants to become a member but you're busy so she leaves. Oh well, it's only $10 per month lost right? Now what if you make that decision 500 times in a month? 500 people try to become members but you don't bother with them because they only equal $10 each. But of course if you had taken each one seriously and worked to have them join your gym, then a month later you'd have $5,000.

It's the same principle. If you fail a single moment, that's all it is. One failed moment. Focus on how badly it makes you feel. Now take on the next moment with that new information fresh in your mind. Don't bury your head in the sand, learn from this! Tell yourself, "I convinced myself to fail in that moment and now I feel bad about it". Stop tricking yourself. You have a monster in your head that is addicted to those sugars and it will do anything it can to trick you into giving into your cravings. Fight the monster.

Do not tell yourself that since you failed one moment you may as well fail all the following moments. It all adds up. Look back at that piece of cake you ate and be proud that instead of falling down a rabbit hole of binging, you just moved on and succeeded with every other moment.

A note about friends:

Your friends and family will try to convince you to cheat, and ultimately to fail. Why? Because your success reflects badly on their own failures. It's just human nature. So they might belittle your efforts or tempt you with treats or do anything they can to derail your efforts, without even being consciously aware that they're doing it. Don't let them. Practice smiling and saying 'no thanks'.

Don't be the person who gives in and eats the cake along with your friends. Don't forget if they could all take a pill tomorrow that would make them lose weight overnight, they all would; in fact, it's been my experience that most people dream of that miracle.

Succeed instead. Do it differently this time. 500 moments from now you will show up and blow them away with how you have transformed yourself. Motivate them! It was only 500 moments and you intend to do 10,000 more because you're now living proof of what a healthy lifestyle can do.

All those snacks and garbage foods you DIDN'T have over the past 2 months have all added up to who you are today and who you're going to be from now on.

Your friends and family will be inspired by your change. They've spent the past 2 months saying 'what's the point of life without cake' and now they'll see the real truth: what's the point of trading your best *self* for a piece of fucking cake?

CHAPTER 6: A FINAL NOTE

This is all about creating a new baseline for your body. After the 500, you can enjoy treats every now and then because that's the realistic way to do this for life.

Do this. When you find yourself making excuses *not* to do this just remember that's how you've been living your life this entire time. That way of thinking has brought you to researching weight loss solutions because you're tired of living like this.

So change the cycle. This isn't difficult. This is a mindset. You don't need any special powers, or an easier job, or to be rich in order to do this. You eat every day. Eat better, 500 times in a row.

These 2 months are going to go by no matter what you do.

Let go of your expectations of immediate change and transformation. This is a lifestyle marathon, not a sprint. Imagine this: A group of millionaires tell you that getting rich is very simple and will only take two months. All you need to do, they tell you, is to follow their steps every day and on the final day you will have a million dollars. After the first few days you look at your bank account and wow you already have $5,000! This is great and you feel great and you're really making progress and you're so excited for your future and for your life again; you've taken control! But, after a week or so you check your bank account and you're still at $5,000. A week later and you're only at $6,000. You should be happy that you made $6,000 in a couple weeks but instead you're wondering how you're ever going to get to one million at this rate. Another two weeks go by and you check your bank account and you're at $25,000. That's a lot of money to make in one month but not even close to enough to become a millionaire in the next 30 days! So, you kind of stick to the program, cheating here and there with the instructions and notice that you're really not making anymore money. Some days you make a couple bucks but then you cheat the program and lose that couple bucks.

Now you feel defeated and wonder what's the point of any of this? You'd rather just take the $25,000 you made and buy a car. So you do just that and now you're back where you started and you tell yourself that some day in the future you'll try again. It wasn't your fault; it just didn't work for you because…reasons.

But what you don't know is two things:

1.   You should have taken time to be proud of yourself for making $25,000 in a month! And you certainly didn't need to blow it all just because you gave up.

2.   If you had believed in yourself and taken pride in every dollar earned, you would have woken up on day 50 with a million dollars in your bank account.

There is no dark secret about getting in great shape that only rich celebrities know. And everybody can do it. You just need to be consistent in your approach, accept that it wont happen overnight and enjoy the frigging process!

Remember this: with every 'before-and-after' picture there are hundreds of pictures in between that on their own look like no change at all. Do this for yourself and stick to this for yourself. Eat. Just eat smart.

Stop trading seconds of happiness for years of disappointment. You can do this. Pick a date and start. This is it.

Don't get bogged down in diet trends or certain foods.
Common sense always prevails.

Food Options

Decision Moment One: Breakfast

- Eggs. Whole eggs. Arguably the perfect food.

- Avocado. Don't be afraid of healthy fats

- Steel Cut Oats with Cinnamon

Decision Moment Two: AM Snack

- Small bunch of mixed nuts

- Cheese and deli meats (no crackers or carbs)

- Cucumber salad

- Coffee with extra cream

Decision Moment: Lunch

- Chicken breast cut into a salad of spinach, cheese, nuts, olive oil, salt, cucumber and tomato (throw it all in a big Tupperware; it's so easy and filling)

- Strips of thin steak with green and red peppers and shredded cheese and parmesan cheese (again, don't be afraid of healthy fats! Its the excess carbs and sugars that we need to worry about)

- Omelette with cheese and asparagus and a handful of mixed nuts (almonds, Brazil, macadamia)

- Sweet Potato, Chicken breast with salsa and green beans

Decision Moment: PM Snack

- Cut up cheeses and apple slices with cinnamon

- Avocado cut up and mixed with shredded cheese

Decision Moment: Dinner

- Fish (cod, salmon) with green beans and brown rice and a couple pieces of cheese (fats keep you full)

- Chicken or steak with parmesan cheese, olive oil, butter, asparagus or broccoli

- Stir fry with meats, veggies, and pumpkin seeds. Drizzle with olive oil and cook with butter

- Chicken thighs with skin on and seasoned salt roasted in the oven and then broiled slightly. Side with a big salad of spinach cucumber tomato red pepper and shredded cheese.

Decision Moment: Evening Temptation or the Long Goodnight

- Sliced up deli meats, pickle, cheese

- Spoonful of Peanut Butter

- Some cottage cheese

- Egg white omelet with red pepper

TIP

- Rule: All drinks must contain 0g Sugar. Get some flavoured carbonated water to address your cravings for pops and juices. You won't miss the crappy drinks after a day or two and you'll sleep so much better!

The Ketogenic Diet and why it works for me (and may for you too)

The Ketogenic diet changed my life. I stopped craving sugars and carbs, felt better and got more results from my workouts. But I don't stay on it all the time. I "re-feed" every couple of weeks with carbs like sweet potatoes and brown rice and steel cut oats.

Here's how it works: You eat mainly healthy fats in each meal with protein and very little carbs. Less than 20grams per day. So for instance, my only carbs come from vegetables when I'm eating Keto.

Why it works: When your body is depleted of carbohydrates it creates energy from your body's stored fat cells. The conversion process creates Ketones as a bi-product as it travels out of the liver and these keynotes take over as the main fuel source for your brain.

So you're using stored fat for fuel and at the same time not taking in any carbs (which would be converting into glucose and stored as fat) nor any sugar. So it's a double hit of converting fat to energy and not creating any new fat cells.

Why it works for me: Eating so much healthy fats keeps me always satiated. I'm never hungry or craving bad carbs. I also love eating cheese and sliced meats as a snack at night so I don't ever feel deprived. It's why it's the only diet I could maintain as a lifestyle.

I eat so many great and full foods, it's easy. If this sounds like something that would work for you too then I encourage you to research the diet and maybe even ask your doctor about it.

A **Low Carb** diet is essentially the same idea except that your protein is not as limited as it is on the ketogenic diet and your fat intake is not as high.

Intermittent Fasting

Intermittent Fasting (IF) is pretty popular at the time of this writing. There are numerous health benefits to fasting as well as stories of successful fat loss using this method. Do your research, try it out for a week and find out if it's right for you!

The beautiful thing about IF is that once you start it's very simple to get used to.

The idea is to go for long periods without eating. So the easiest way to do this is to incorporate the time you are sleeping and already not eating anyways. So if you just eat between, say, 12pm and 9pm then you'll be fasting for 15 hours every day. It's very simple to do once you decide to do it.

If you can incorporate some "fasted cardio"- performing a cardiovascular activity while in a fasted state- then the theory is that you will be using stored calories as a fuel source instead of the food you just took in.

Therefore, if you decide to do IF, try to do a workout in the morning before you eat. Even something as simple as jumping rope in your backyard or doing some fast pushups and sit-ups in your bedroom.

Just Remember:

The key to The 500 Solution is focusing on your MIND and in cutting out INDECISION. Do not wonder if you should eat the chips or order the pizza, decide that you won't. DECIDE that you do not get a muffin or cookie with your coffee.

Suffer slightly, it's okay. You will survive not giving in to your every desire. And what's more, you'll be better for it.